UNDERSTANDING ALZHEIMER'S DISEASE

Comprehensive Guide To Symptoms, Diagnosis, Treatment, And Care Strategies For Effective Management And Support

DR. LINCOLN WAYLON

Copyright © [2024] [Lincoln Waylon]. All Rights Reserved.

The copyright laws of the United States of America and other nations safeguard this publication. Except for brief quotations included in critical reviews and certain other non-commercial uses allowed by copyright law, no part of this book may be reproduced, distributed, or transmitted in any form or by any means, including photocopying, recording, or other electronic or mechanical methods, without the prior written permission of the copyright owner.

DISCLAIMER

This book contains information that should only be used for educational and informational reasons; it is not meant to be used as a source of medical or psychological advice. The author's studies, life experiences, and expertise in the area of health and wellness served as the foundation for the content. It should not, however, be used in place of expert counsel, a diagnosis, or medical care.

Any queries you may have about a physical or mental health issue should always be directed toward the advice of a licensed healthcare provider or mental health specialist. With regard to the efficacy or outcomes of the methods or suggestions included in this book, the author and publisher make no representations or warranties.

Any information or methods in this book are used entirely at the reader's own risk and discretion. The material provided here may be used or misused, and neither the author nor the publisher will be held responsible for any results, losses, or negative impacts.

Keep in mind that everyone has different demands and reactions to health and wellness routines. Any health and wellness plans you implement must be customized to your particular circumstances, and you should speak with experts to make sure the plans meet your needs.

TABLE OF CONTENTS

CHAPTER ONE 13
   OVERVIEW OF ALZHEIMER'S DISEASE 13
      DEFINITION AND HISTORY 13
      KEY STATISTICS AND IMPACT 14
      COMMON SYMPTOMS AND STAGES 15
      DIFFERENTIATING ALZHEIMER'S FROM OTHER TYPES OF 16
      IMPORTANCE OF EARLY INTERVENTION 18

CHAPTER TWO 19
   CAUSES AND RISK FACTORS 19
      GENETIC PREDISPOSITIONS 19
      ENVIRONMENTAL AND LIFESTYLE FACTORS 20
      ROLE OF AGE AND FAMILY HISTORY 22
      OTHER HEALTH CONDITIONS INFLUENCING RISK 23
      ONGOING RESEARCH AND THEORIES 24

CHAPTER THREE 27
   HOW ALZHEIMER'S AFFECTS THE BRAIN 27
      BRAIN STRUCTURE CHANGES 27
      FORMATION OF AMYLOID PLAQUES AND TAU TANGLES 28
      IMPACT ON NEURON FUNCTION 30
      COGNITIVE DECLINE AND MEMORY LOSS 31
      NEUROLOGICAL PATHWAYS AFFECTED 32

CHAPTER FOUR 35
   DIAGNOSING ALZHEIMER'S DISEASE 35
      DIAGNOSTIC CRITERIA AND GUIDELINES 35

    COMMON DIAGNOSTIC TESTS AND PROCEDURES 36
    ROLE OF IMAGING TECHNIQUES..38
    EVALUATING SYMPTOMS AND COGNITIVE FUNCTION.............39
    IMPORTANCE OF RULING OUT OTHER CONDITIONS 41

CHAPTER FIVE..43
  TREATMENT OPTIONS AND THERAPIES 43
    OVERVIEW OF FDA-APPROVED MEDICATIONS 43
    POTENTIAL BENEFITS AND SIDE EFFECTS...................................44
    NON-DRUG THERAPIES AND LIFESTYLE CHANGES 45
    ROLE OF CLINICAL TRIALS AND RESEARCH STUDIES 46
    INTEGRATING TREATMENTS INTO DAILY LIFE.............................47

CHAPTER SIX..49
  MANAGING SYMPTOMS AND COMPLICATIONS 49
    STRATEGIES FOR MEMORY AND COGNITIVE SUPPORT 49
    MANAGING BEHAVIORAL AND PSYCHOLOGICAL SYMPTOMS...........50
    APPROACHES TO DAILY LIVING CHALLENGES 52
    SUPPORT FOR PHYSICAL HEALTH ISSUES 53
    IMPORTANCE OF ROUTINE AND STRUCTURE..............................55

CHAPTER SEVEN 57
  THE ROLE OF CAREGIVERS AND FAMILY SUPPORT 57
    RESPONSIBILITIES AND CHALLENGES OF CAREGIVING 57
    TECHNIQUES FOR EFFECTIVE CAREGIVING 58
    IMPORTANCE OF CAREGIVER SELF-CARE 59
    RESOURCES AND SUPPORT NETWORKS......................................60
    COMMUNICATING WITH HEALTHCARE PROFESSIONALS 61

CHAPTER EIGHT 63

LEGAL AND FINANCIAL CONSIDERATIONS 63

PLANNING FOR FUTURE CARE NEEDS 63
MANAGING FINANCES AND LEGAL DOCUMENTS 64
UNDERSTANDING INSURANCE AND BENEFITS 66
LEGAL RIGHTS AND PROTECTIONS FOR INDIVIDUALS WITH 67
RESOURCES FOR LEGAL AND FINANCIAL ADVICE 69

CHAPTER NINE 71

LIVING WITH ALZHEIMER'S DISEASE 71

ADAPTING TO CHANGES IN LIFESTYLE 71
ENSURING SAFETY AND COMFORT 72
ENGAGING IN MEANINGFUL ACTIVITIES 74
BUILDING A SUPPORT NETWORK 75
PLANNING FOR END-OF-LIFE CARE 76

CHAPTER TEN 79

FAQS 79

WHAT ARE THE EARLY SIGNS OF ALZHEIMER'S DISEASE? 79
ARE THERE ANY LIFESTYLE CHANGES THAT CAN REDUCE THE 80
HOW IS ALZHEIMER'S DISEASE DIAGNOSED? 81
WHAT TYPES OF MEDICATIONS ARE USED TO TREAT 82
HOW CAN CAREGIVERS COPE WITH THE CHALLENGES OF CARING ... 84

ABOUT THE BOOK

Understanding Alzheimer's disease is a vital resource for anyone seeking to grasp the complexities of this challenging condition. The book begins with a comprehensive overview, offering a clear definition and historical context of Alzheimer's, alongside key statistics that highlight its significant impact on individuals and society. It delves into the common symptoms and stages of the disease, providing a crucial distinction between Alzheimer's and other types of dementia. This foundational knowledge emphasizes the importance of early intervention, which can significantly influence the course of the disease and the quality of life for those affected.

The exploration of causes and risk factors presents a thorough examination of genetic predispositions, environmental and lifestyle factors, and the roles of age and family history. By addressing these elements, the book sheds light on how various health conditions can influence the risk of developing Alzheimer's, while also presenting the latest research and theories in the field. This section equips readers with an understanding of the multifaceted nature of Alzheimer's, contributing to a deeper awareness of its origins and risk factors.

The book's discussion on how Alzheimer's affects the brain provides an in-depth look at the structural changes that occur, including the formation of amyloid plaques and tau tangles. It explains the impact on neuron function, cognitive decline, and memory loss, as well as the neurological pathways that are affected. This detailed analysis is essential for comprehending how Alzheimer's impairs brain function and affects daily life.

Diagnosing Alzheimer's Disease is addressed with a focus on the diagnostic criteria and guidelines that healthcare professionals use. The book covers common diagnostic tests and procedures, including imaging techniques, and highlights the importance of evaluating symptoms and cognitive function. By emphasizing the need to rule out other conditions, the book underscores the complexity of an accurate diagnosis and the role it plays in effective management.

Treatment options and therapies are thoroughly examined, offering an overview of FDA-approved medications, their potential benefits and side effects, and non-drug therapies. The discussion extends to lifestyle changes and the role of clinical trials and research studies in advancing treatment options. This section provides practical guidance on integrating various treatments into daily life to support individuals with Alzheimer's.

Managing symptoms and complications are addressed with strategies for supporting memory and cognitive function, managing behavioral and psychological symptoms, and tackling daily living challenges.

The book also covers the importance of routine and structure, which are crucial for maintaining quality of life for both individuals with Alzheimer's and their caregivers.

The role of caregivers and family support is highlighted, focusing on the responsibilities and challenges of caregiving, effective caregiving techniques, and the importance of caregiver self-care. The book provides resources and support networks, as well as guidance on communicating with healthcare professionals, which are essential for those supporting loved ones with Alzheimer's.

Legal and financial considerations are explored in detail, offering advice on planning for future care needs, managing finances and legal documents, and understanding insurance and benefits. The book also addresses the legal rights and protections for individuals with Alzheimer's, providing resources for legal and financial advice to ensure informed decision-making.

Living with Alzheimer's disease is discussed with a focus on adapting to lifestyle changes, ensuring safety and comfort, engaging in meaningful activities, and building a support network. The book also emphasizes the importance of planning for end-of-life care, addressing the emotional and practical aspects of living with Alzheimer's.

Throughout, the book provides answers to frequently asked questions about early signs of Alzheimer's, lifestyle changes that may reduce risk, diagnostic procedures, treatment options, and caregiver coping strategies. This comprehensive approach ensures that readers are well-informed and equipped to navigate the complexities of Alzheimer's disease.

CHAPTER ONE
OVERVIEW OF ALZHEIMER'S DISEASE
DEFINITION AND HISTORY

Alzheimer's disease is a progressive neurodegenerative disorder that primarily affects memory, thinking, and behavior. It is the most common form of dementia, characterized by the gradual decline of cognitive functions due to damage to brain cells. The disease was first described by Dr. Alois Alzheimer in 1906, after whom it is named, following his observations of a patient with peculiar symptoms and brain abnormalities post-mortem. The defining features of Alzheimer's are the accumulation of amyloid plaques and neurofibrillary tangles in the brain, which disrupt neuronal communication and lead to cell death.

Historically, Alzheimer's disease was considered rare, but its prevalence has significantly increased with the aging global population.

As people live longer, the number of individuals diagnosed with Alzheimer's has risen, making it a major public health issue. Research into Alzheimer's has evolved over the years, shifting from a focus on symptom management to exploring underlying causes, potential risk factors, and more effective treatments. Understanding the history of Alzheimer's helps in appreciating the advancements in research and the ongoing efforts to combat this debilitating disease.

KEY STATISTICS AND IMPACT

Alzheimer's disease affects approximately 6.7 million Americans aged 65 and older, with projections indicating that this number will nearly double by 2050 due to an aging population. Globally, over 50 million people are living with dementia and Alzheimer's accounts for 60-70% of these cases. The impact of Alzheimer's extends beyond the individual, placing a significant emotional and financial burden on families and caregivers.

The annual cost of Alzheimer's care in the United States is estimated to exceed $355 billion, including direct medical costs and unpaid care provided by family members.

The societal impact of Alzheimer's disease is profound, affecting not just the individuals diagnosed but also their families and communities. As the disease progresses, it often leads to increased dependency, requiring extensive care and support. This can result in a strain on healthcare systems and a need for specialized services, highlighting the importance of support systems and resources for both patients and caregivers. Understanding these statistics underscores the urgency of advancing research and improving care strategies.

COMMON SYMPTOMS AND STAGES

Alzheimer's disease typically progresses through several stages, each with distinct symptoms. In the early stage, individuals may experience mild memory loss, confusion about time or place, and difficulty with complex tasks. As the disease advances to the moderate stage, symptoms become more pronounced, including significant memory loss, confusion about personal history, and difficulty recognizing familiar people. This stage often involves behavioral changes, such as increased agitation or withdrawal from social activities.

In the late stage of Alzheimer's, individuals lose the ability to communicate effectively and may require full-time care. Symptoms include severe memory loss, an inability to recognize loved ones, and a loss of physical abilities such as walking or swallowing. This stage is characterized by a profound decline in cognitive functions, making it challenging for patients to engage in daily activities and requiring extensive care and support from family members or caregivers.

DIFFERENTIATING ALZHEIMER'S FROM OTHER TYPES OF DEMENTIA

Differentiating Alzheimer's disease from other forms of dementia is crucial for accurate diagnosis and effective treatment. While Alzheimer's is the most common type, other dementias, such as vascular dementia, frontotemporal dementia, and Lewy body dementia, present with different symptoms and underlying causes. Vascular dementia often follows a stroke or series of mini-strokes and is characterized by sudden changes in cognitive abilities. Frontotemporal dementia typically involves changes in personality and behavior rather than memory loss.

Lewy body dementia is marked by the presence of abnormal protein deposits called Lewy bodies in the brain, leading to fluctuating cognition, visual hallucinations, and motor symptoms similar to Parkinson's disease. Accurate diagnosis involves a comprehensive assessment of symptoms, medical history, and sometimes neuroimaging or biomarker testing. Understanding these differences is essential for developing a tailored treatment plan and providing the most appropriate care for individuals with dementia.

IMPORTANCE OF EARLY INTERVENTION

Early intervention in Alzheimer's disease is crucial for slowing the progression of symptoms and improving quality of life. Identifying the disease at an early stage allows for the timely management of symptoms through medications, lifestyle changes, and cognitive therapies. Early treatment can help in maintaining cognitive functions for a longer period and managing behavioral symptoms more effectively.

In addition to medical treatments, early intervention includes educating patients and caregivers about the disease, providing access to support services, and planning for future care needs. This proactive approach helps in reducing the impact of the disease on daily living and allows families to make informed decisions about care and support. The importance of early intervention cannot be overstated, as it significantly influences the trajectory of the disease and the overall well-being of those affected.

CHAPTER TWO

CAUSES AND RISK FACTORS

GENETIC PREDISPOSITIONS

Genetic predispositions play a significant role in the development of Alzheimer's disease. Certain genes, such as the APOE ε4 allele, are associated with an increased risk of developing the disease. This gene variant can affect the way amyloid-beta protein is processed in the brain, contributing to the formation of plaques, a hallmark of Alzheimer's.

Testing for these genetic markers can provide insight into an individual's risk level, though having these genes does not guarantee onset but rather indicates a higher susceptibility.

In practical terms, individuals with a family history of Alzheimer's may choose to undergo genetic counseling and testing to understand their risk better. Genetic predisposition tests are usually conducted through blood samples or saliva, and results can guide preventive strategies and lifestyle adjustments. Individuals need to discuss these results with healthcare professionals to develop a personalized approach to monitoring and managing their cognitive health.

Understanding genetic predispositions also involves recognizing that while genes contribute to risk, they interact with environmental and lifestyle factors. This interaction emphasizes the importance of a holistic approach to managing Alzheimer's risk, combining genetic information with proactive lifestyle choices and medical supervision.

ENVIRONMENTAL AND LIFESTYLE FACTORS

Environmental and lifestyle factors significantly impact the risk of developing Alzheimer's disease. Factors such as diet, physical activity, and exposure to environmental toxins can influence brain health over time. For example, a diet high in fruits, vegetables, and healthy fats, like the Mediterranean diet, is associated with a lower risk of cognitive decline. Regular physical exercise helps maintain cardiovascular health, which is crucial for optimal brain function.

Practical steps to mitigate risk include adopting a balanced diet rich in antioxidants and omega-3 fatty acids and engaging in consistent physical activity. Incorporating activities such as walking, swimming, or strength training into daily routines can enhance overall brain health.

Additionally, minimizing exposure to environmental pollutants and toxins by using air purifiers and avoiding smoking can contribute to long-term cognitive health.

Adopting a mentally stimulating lifestyle also plays a role. Engaging in activities that challenge the brain, such as learning new skills, solving puzzles, or participating in social activities, can help maintain cognitive function. These lifestyle choices, when practiced regularly, can serve as preventative measures against Alzheimer's disease.

ROLE OF AGE AND FAMILY HISTORY

Age and family history are fundamental factors in understanding Alzheimer's risk. As people age, the likelihood of developing Alzheimer's increases, with the majority of cases occurring in individuals over 65. Age-related changes in brain structure and function, such as reduced blood flow and neuronal loss, contribute to the higher incidence of Alzheimer's in older adults.

Family history further compounds the risk, especially if multiple relatives have been diagnosed with Alzheimer's. Inherited genetic mutations, particularly those found in early-onset Alzheimer's, can cause the disease to appear before the age of 65. For families with a history of early-onset Alzheimer's, genetic counseling and testing can help identify risks and inform monitoring strategies.

Practical approaches for those concerned about age and family history include regular cognitive assessments and proactive lifestyle adjustments.

Keeping track of changes in memory and cognitive abilities and discussing these with healthcare providers can lead to early detection and management strategies.

Additionally, maintaining a healthy lifestyle, as mentioned previously, remains crucial for mitigating risks associated with aging and family history.

OTHER HEALTH CONDITIONS INFLUENCING RISK

Other health conditions can influence the risk of developing Alzheimer's disease. Conditions such as diabetes, hypertension, and high cholesterol are linked to an increased risk of cognitive decline. Diabetes, for instance, can lead to increased inflammation and oxidative stress, which negatively impact brain health. Similarly, untreated hypertension can damage blood vessels in the brain, affecting cognitive function.

Managing these health conditions through medication, diet, and lifestyle changes is vital.

Individuals with diabetes should work closely with their healthcare providers to control blood sugar levels, while those with hypertension should monitor blood pressure and adhere to prescribed treatments. A heart-healthy diet low in saturated fats and high in fiber can help manage cholesterol levels and reduce overall risk.

Routine health check-ups and preventive measures are key in addressing these conditions. Regular monitoring of blood sugar, blood pressure, and cholesterol levels can prevent complications and reduce the risk of Alzheimer's disease.

Effective management of these conditions contributes to overall brain health and lowers the likelihood of cognitive decline.

ONGOING RESEARCH AND THEORIES

Ongoing research continues to explore the causes and mechanisms behind Alzheimer's disease. Scientists are investigating the roles of amyloid plaques and tau tangles in the brain, with studies focusing on how these proteins contribute to neuronal damage and cognitive decline.

Researchers are also exploring the impact of neuroinflammation and genetic interactions on the disease's progression.

Emerging theories include the role of the gut-brain axis and its influence on Alzheimer's. Research suggests that gut health and microbiota composition might affect brain health and inflammation, potentially linking digestive health to cognitive function.

Additionally, there is growing interest in the role of sleep disturbances in Alzheimer's risk, with studies examining how poor sleep quality may accelerate disease onset.

Practical involvement in research includes participating in clinical trials and staying informed about new findings. Individuals interested in contributing to the understanding of Alzheimer's can explore opportunities to enroll in studies or support research initiatives. Staying engaged with the latest research developments helps individuals make informed decisions about their health and preventive measures.

CHAPTER THREE

HOW ALZHEIMER'S AFFECTS THE BRAIN

BRAIN STRUCTURE CHANGES

Alzheimer's disease brings significant changes to the brain's structure, starting with the shrinkage of specific brain regions. The hippocampus, crucial for forming new memories, experiences noticeable atrophy early in the disease, which impairs the ability to retain new information. As Alzheimer's progresses, the shrinkage extends to other areas, including the cortex, which is involved in higher cognitive functions such as reasoning and planning. This progressive loss of brain tissue results in a reduction of overall brain volume, observable in imaging scans.

The atrophy is due to the loss of neurons and their connections, which are essential for communication within the brain. The damage to these structures is linked to the disease's hallmark features: amyloid plaques and tau tangles.

The destruction of neural networks disrupts the brain's ability to process and integrate information efficiently, contributing to the cognitive decline observed in individuals with Alzheimer's.

These structural changes not only impact memory and cognitive functions but also affect daily life activities.

The ongoing brain deterioration leads to challenges in carrying out routine tasks and makes it increasingly difficult for individuals to manage their environment and personal needs independently.

FORMATION OF AMYLOID PLAQUES AND TAU TANGLES

Amyloid plaques and tau tangles are two key pathological features of Alzheimer's disease. Amyloid plaques are abnormal clusters of protein fragments, primarily beta-amyloid, that accumulate between nerve cells. These plaques disrupt cell-to-cell communication, leading to inflammation and eventual cell death.

Their presence is a critical marker in diagnosing Alzheimer's and understanding its progression.

Tau tangles are formed from hyperphosphorylated tau proteins, which aggregate inside neurons, creating twisted fibers. These tangles interfere with the transport system within neurons, essential for nutrient and waste removal.

As tau tangles accumulate, they contribute to the breakdown of the neuron's internal structure, exacerbating the loss of neural function and cell death.

The formation of both plaques and tangles starts in specific brain regions and spreads over time, correlating with the severity of cognitive symptoms. The presence and distribution of these pathological features provide insights into the disease's progression and help in developing targeted therapies to combat their effects.

IMPACT ON NEURON FUNCTION

Alzheimer's disease significantly impacts neuron function by disrupting the communication pathways between brain cells. Healthy neurons rely on complex signaling mechanisms to transmit information effectively. However, the accumulation of amyloid plaques impairs these signals, leading to reduced efficiency in information transfer and synaptic function.

Tau tangles further compound this issue by obstructing the neuron's internal transport system. This disruption prevents essential molecules and nutrients from reaching their destination within the cell, causing metabolic imbalances and impairing neuronal health. As neurons lose their ability to communicate and maintain themselves, they become increasingly vulnerable to damage and eventual death.

The decline in neuron function is directly related to the cognitive deficits experienced in Alzheimer's. As the disease progresses, the widespread damage to neural circuits impairs memory, reasoning, and other cognitive abilities, making daily activities and independent living increasingly challenging.

COGNITIVE DECLINE AND MEMORY LOSS

Cognitive decline and memory loss are among the most noticeable symptoms of Alzheimer's disease. The early stages often involve difficulties in forming new memories and retaining recent information. Individuals may struggle to recall names, events, or newly learned facts, which can lead to frustration and confusion.

As Alzheimer's advances, the cognitive decline becomes more pronounced, affecting both short-term and long-term memory. People may forget significant life events, conversations, or appointments, and may have trouble recognizing familiar faces or navigating previously known environments. This progressive memory loss impacts daily functioning, making it difficult for individuals to maintain their independence.

The decline in cognitive functions also affects other mental processes, including reasoning, problem-solving, and judgment. These changes can lead to difficulties in managing finances, planning activities, and performing routine tasks, further diminishing the quality of life for those affected.

NEUROLOGICAL PATHWAYS AFFECTED

Alzheimer's disease affects several crucial neurological pathways that are responsible for cognitive functions. The disease disrupts the cholinergic system, which relies on neurotransmitters like acetylcholine for memory and learning.

The loss of cholinergic neurons in the brain contributes to the cognitive deficits observed in Alzheimer's patients.

Additionally, Alzheimer's impacts the brain's default mode network, a network of regions that is active during rest and introspection. Disruption in this network affects self-referential thinking and memory consolidation, further impairing cognitive functions. As the disease progresses, these disruptions become more widespread, affecting various brain regions involved in processing and integrating information.

The widespread damage to neurological pathways results in the impairment of essential cognitive and memory functions. Understanding which pathways are affected helps in developing targeted treatments that aim to preserve or restore function, potentially slowing the progression of the disease and improving the quality of life for those affected.

CHAPTER FOUR

DIAGNOSING ALZHEIMER'S DISEASE

DIAGNOSTIC CRITERIA AND GUIDELINES

To diagnose Alzheimer's disease, clinicians follow established diagnostic criteria, primarily outlined by the National Institute on Aging-Alzheimer's Association (NIA-AA). These guidelines emphasize a thorough patient history and clinical assessment to identify symptoms consistent with Alzheimer's disease.

Key diagnostic criteria include the presence of cognitive decline, particularly in memory, and the impact of these symptoms on daily functioning. Clinicians use a combination of criteria, including the gradual onset of symptoms and their progression over time, to confirm the diagnosis.

Diagnostic guidelines also involve assessing biomarkers through cerebrospinal fluid (CSF) analysis or blood tests, which can reveal amyloid-beta plaques and tau proteins characteristic of Alzheimer's. These biomarkers, alongside clinical symptoms, provide a comprehensive view of the disease's presence and progression. Adhering to these guidelines ensures a standardized approach to diagnosing Alzheimer's, minimizing the risk of misdiagnosis and improving the accuracy of the results.

It is crucial for clinicians to continually update their knowledge of diagnostic criteria and guidelines, as advances in research may refine or introduce new standards. Regular training and staying informed about the latest developments in Alzheimer's diagnostics contribute to maintaining diagnostic accuracy and ensuring patients receive appropriate care based on the most current evidence.

COMMON DIAGNOSTIC TESTS AND PROCEDURES

The diagnosis of Alzheimer's disease commonly involves several diagnostic tests and procedures to confirm the presence of the disease and assess its severity. Cognitive testing is one of the primary methods, where standardized tools such as the Mini-Mental State Examination (MMSE) or the Montreal Cognitive Assessment (MoCA) are used to evaluate memory, attention, language, and executive function. These tests help establish the extent of cognitive decline and track changes over time.

Neuropsychological assessments provide a more in-depth evaluation, assessing various cognitive domains to distinguish Alzheimer's from other types of dementia. These tests can be detailed and time-consuming but are essential for a comprehensive diagnosis. In addition to cognitive tests, clinicians may use laboratory tests to rule out other causes of cognitive decline, such as vitamin deficiencies or thyroid disorders, which can present with similar symptoms but are treatable if identified.

Another critical component of diagnosis is patient and family interviews to understand the onset and progression of symptoms. These interviews provide context to the cognitive tests and help clinicians differentiate Alzheimer's disease from other conditions with similar presentations. Combining these various diagnostic tools ensures a thorough assessment and accurate diagnosis of Alzheimer's disease.

ROLE OF IMAGING TECHNIQUES

Imaging techniques play a crucial role in the diagnosis of Alzheimer's disease, providing visual insights into brain changes associated with the condition. Magnetic Resonance Imaging (MRI) is frequently used to identify structural brain changes, such as atrophy in the hippocampus, which is often seen in Alzheimer's patients. MRI can help visualize the extent of brain damage and monitor changes over time.

Positron Emission Tomography (PET) scans are another essential imaging technique, used to detect amyloid-beta plaques and tau tangles, which are hallmark features of Alzheimer's disease. PET imaging provides a detailed view of these pathological features, aiding in the differentiation of Alzheimer's from other types of dementia. Additionally, PET scans can help assess brain metabolism and function, offering a comprehensive perspective on how the disease affects the brain.

Functional imaging techniques, such as Functional MRI (fMRI) or Single Photon Emission Computed Tomography (SPECT), can also be employed to assess brain activity and blood flow. These imaging methods help clinicians understand the impact of Alzheimer's on brain function, which can be useful in diagnosing and monitoring disease progression. Together, these imaging techniques provide valuable information that supports accurate diagnosis and effective management of Alzheimer's disease.

EVALUATING SYMPTOMS AND COGNITIVE FUNCTION

Evaluating symptoms and cognitive function is a critical aspect of diagnosing Alzheimer's disease, as it provides insights into the severity and progression of the condition.

Clinicians conduct a comprehensive evaluation of cognitive functions, including memory, language, attention, and problem-solving skills, to assess how these functions are impacted by the disease. This evaluation typically involves structured interviews and standardized tests designed to quantify cognitive deficits and track changes over time.

Observations of daily living activities and functional abilities are also essential for understanding the impact of cognitive decline on a patient's quality of life. Assessments may include evaluating the patient's ability to perform routine tasks, manage finances, or handle personal care.

This functional assessment helps determine the level of impairment and informs care planning and support needs.

The evaluation process needs to involve both the patient and their caregivers, as caregivers can provide valuable insights into changes in behavior, personality, and daily functioning that may not be immediately apparent during clinical assessments. This comprehensive approach ensures a more accurate understanding of the patient's condition and helps tailor interventions to their specific needs.

IMPORTANCE OF RULING OUT OTHER CONDITIONS

Ruling out other conditions is a crucial step in diagnosing Alzheimer's disease, as several other medical and psychological conditions can mimic its symptoms. Conditions such as depression, anxiety, and thyroid disorders can present with cognitive decline and memory problems similar to those seen in Alzheimer's. Comprehensive testing and evaluation are necessary to differentiate Alzheimer's from these other conditions to ensure appropriate diagnosis and treatment.

Clinicians conduct various tests to exclude other potential causes of cognitive impairment, including blood tests, imaging studies, and neurological evaluations. For instance, checking thyroid function or vitamin levels can identify deficiencies that might be contributing to cognitive issues. Additionally, neuropsychological testing can help distinguish between Alzheimer's and other types of dementia, such as vascular dementia or frontotemporal dementia.

A thorough medical history and assessment of the patient's overall health are also vital in this process. By systematically ruling out other conditions, clinicians can confirm the diagnosis of Alzheimer's disease and develop a targeted treatment plan that addresses the specific needs of the patient. This meticulous approach helps ensure that patients receive the most accurate diagnosis and effective care.

CHAPTER FIVE
TREATMENT OPTIONS AND THERAPIES
OVERVIEW OF FDA-APPROVED MEDICATIONS

FDA-approved medications for Alzheimer's disease primarily include cholinesterase inhibitors and NMDA receptor antagonists. Cholinesterase inhibitors, such as donepezil, rivastigmine, and galantamine, work by increasing levels of acetylcholine in the brain, a neurotransmitter associated with memory and learning.

NMDA receptor antagonists like memantine help regulate the activity of glutamate, another neurotransmitter involved in brain function. These medications can help manage symptoms and potentially slow the progression of the disease.

Patients typically start with a low dose of these medications, gradually increasing as tolerated, to minimize side effects and monitor efficacy. The choice of medication and dosage depends on individual health factors, such as the severity of symptoms and any co-existing medical conditions. Regular follow-up appointments are essential to adjust treatment plans based on patient response and side effects.

POTENTIAL BENEFITS AND SIDE EFFECTS

The primary benefit of cholinesterase inhibitors is their potential to improve cognitive function and daily living activities, enhancing quality of life. For some individuals, these medications may delay the progression of symptoms and support better management of cognitive decline. However, side effects can occur, including nausea, diarrhea, insomnia, and muscle cramps. Patients and caregivers need to report any adverse effects to the healthcare provider for proper management and potential adjustments in treatment.

NMDA receptor antagonists may provide additional benefits for patients with moderate to severe Alzheimer's by improving memory and cognitive functions. Side effects may include dizziness, headache, and constipation. As with cholinesterase inhibitors, careful monitoring and communication with healthcare professionals are crucial to balance benefits with manageable side effects.

NON-DRUG THERAPIES AND LIFESTYLE CHANGES

Non-drug therapies and lifestyle changes play a critical role in managing Alzheimer's disease. Cognitive stimulation therapy, which involves engaging in activities that stimulate mental functioning, can help improve cognitive abilities and maintain daily skills. Physical exercise, such as walking or swimming, is also beneficial as it promotes overall health and may slow cognitive decline.

Regular social interaction and mental activities, like puzzles or reading, help keep the brain active and engaged.

Dietary changes, including a balanced diet rich in antioxidants and omega-3 fatty acids, can support brain health.

A Mediterranean-style diet, for instance, is often recommended for its potential benefits in reducing cognitive decline. Additionally, maintaining a structured routine and creating a supportive environment helps individuals manage daily tasks and reduces stress, which can further aid in symptom management.

ROLE OF CLINICAL TRIALS AND RESEARCH STUDIES

Clinical trials and research studies are vital for advancing treatments for Alzheimer's disease. These studies test new medications, therapies, and approaches to improve patient outcomes and understand the disease better.

Participation in clinical trials can provide access to cutting-edge treatments and contribute to the development of future therapies. Individuals interested in participating should consult their healthcare providers to explore suitable trials and understand the potential benefits and risks involved.

Research studies also focus on understanding the underlying mechanisms of Alzheimer's and identifying biomarkers for early diagnosis. Staying informed about ongoing research can provide insights into emerging treatments and offer hope for future advancements. Healthcare providers often have information about current trials and can guide patients and families through the process of participating in research studies.

INTEGRATING TREATMENTS INTO DAILY LIFE

Integrating treatments into daily life requires a comprehensive approach to ensure effective management of Alzheimer's symptoms. Medication adherence is crucial; setting reminders or using pill organizers can help patients stay on track with their prescriptions.

Establishing a daily routine that incorporates cognitive exercises, physical activity, and social interaction supports overall well-being and helps manage symptoms.

Incorporating supportive tools and strategies, such as memory aids, labels, and simplified routines, can assist individuals in maintaining independence and managing daily tasks. Caregivers play a key role in providing support, creating a structured environment, and monitoring the effectiveness of treatments. Regular communication with healthcare professionals ensures that treatment plans are adjusted as needed and that both patients and caregivers are supported throughout the journey.

CHAPTER SIX

MANAGING SYMPTOMS AND COMPLICATIONS

STRATEGIES FOR MEMORY AND COGNITIVE SUPPORT

To support memory and cognitive function in individuals with Alzheimer's disease, it's essential to use strategies that cater to their changing needs. Techniques such as creating a consistent environment and using memory aids can significantly improve daily functioning. Implementing tools like calendars, reminder notes, and digital devices can help reinforce memory and assist with daily tasks. Visual cues, such as labeled drawers or doors, also help individuals remember where things are and can simplify their environment.

Engaging in mentally stimulating activities is another key strategy. Puzzles, reading, and brain games can help maintain cognitive function by providing regular mental exercise. Tailoring these activities to the person's interests and abilities ensures they remain engaged and challenged without becoming frustrated. Additionally, incorporating activities that promote social interaction, such as group hobbies or community events, can boost cognitive health by providing both mental stimulation and emotional support.

Establishing routines and consistency in daily activities is crucial. Consistent schedules for meals, medication, and sleep can reduce confusion and anxiety. Breaking tasks into smaller, manageable steps and using checklists can help individuals with Alzheimer's follow through on daily responsibilities. Encouraging family members to participate in these routines can also create a supportive and familiar environment, aiding in memory retention and cognitive stability.

MANAGING BEHAVIORAL AND PSYCHOLOGICAL SYMPTOMS

Behavioral and psychological symptoms, such as aggression, agitation, and depression, are common in Alzheimer's disease and require targeted management strategies. To address these symptoms, it's important to first identify potential triggers, such as changes in routine or environmental factors. Implementing a calm and predictable environment can help minimize agitation and confusion. Ensuring that the person feels safe and comfortable can reduce anxiety and improve overall mood.

Non-pharmacological interventions, such as cognitive-behavioral therapy and reminiscence therapy, can be effective in managing psychological symptoms. Cognitive-behavioral therapy focuses on modifying negative thought patterns and behaviors, while reminiscence therapy uses past experiences and memories to improve mood and emotional well-being. Engaging in these therapeutic approaches can help address symptoms like depression and anxiety in a supportive manner.

In some cases, medication may be necessary to manage severe symptoms. Consulting with a healthcare professional to evaluate the need for medication is important. When prescribed, medications should be carefully monitored for effectiveness and potential side effects. Regular follow-ups with healthcare providers can ensure that any adjustments needed for optimal symptom management are made promptly.

APPROACHES TO DAILY LIVING CHALLENGES

Managing daily living challenges involves adapting environments and routines to enhance independence and safety. For example, modifying home environments with assistive devices such as grab bars in the bathroom and clear labeling of household items can prevent accidents and aid in navigation. Simplifying tasks by organizing daily essentials and using adaptive tools can help individuals with Alzheimer's maintain their independence.

Encouraging participation in daily activities, while considering the individual's abilities, can foster a sense of accomplishment and self-worth. Using step-by-step instructions and visual prompts can assist in completing tasks such as cooking or dressing. Breaking tasks into smaller, more manageable segments can reduce feelings of overwhelm and help maintain engagement in daily routines.

Family members and caregivers play a critical role in supporting daily living. Providing assistance and encouragement while respecting the individual's autonomy can balance support with independence. Open communication with caregivers about the person's preferences and abilities can help tailor daily routines and activities to better suit their needs and improve their quality of life.

SUPPORT FOR PHYSICAL HEALTH ISSUES

Addressing physical health issues in individuals with Alzheimer's involves a comprehensive approach to managing medical conditions and ensuring overall wellness. Regular medical check-ups are essential for monitoring chronic conditions such as diabetes or hypertension. Adhering to prescribed treatments and medications can prevent complications and maintain physical health. Coordinating care with healthcare professionals ensures that all aspects of the individual's health are addressed.

Physical activity is a vital component of managing health in Alzheimer's patients. Engaging in regular exercise tailored to the individual's abilities can improve strength, mobility, and overall well-being. Activities such as walking, stretching, or gentle aerobics can help maintain physical fitness and enhance mood. Creating a structured exercise routine can also provide cognitive benefits by improving circulation and overall brain function.

Nutrition plays a crucial role in physical health management. A balanced diet that includes a variety of fruits, vegetables, whole grains, and lean proteins can support overall health and energy levels. Monitoring dietary intake and adjusting as needed to address specific health concerns, such as weight loss or poor appetite, can improve the individual's nutritional status and overall quality of life.

IMPORTANCE OF ROUTINE AND STRUCTURE

Establishing a daily routine and structure is fundamental for individuals with Alzheimer's disease as it provides a sense of stability and predictability. Consistent routines for daily activities such as meals, medication, and bedtime can help reduce confusion and anxiety. Structured environments with clearly defined schedules can help individuals manage their day more effectively and feel more secure.

Incorporating familiar activities and personal interests into the daily routine can enhance engagement and satisfaction. Allowing the individual to maintain some level of control over their schedule and activities can improve their sense of autonomy and well-being. Adapting routines as needed while maintaining a consistent overall structure can help address changing needs and preferences.

Family members and caregivers should collaborate to create and maintain routines that are realistic and manageable.

Regular communication about the individual's needs and adjustments to their schedule can ensure that routines are effective and supportive. Consistent routines not only assist with daily management but also contribute to a more positive and stable living environment for individuals with Alzheimer's.

CHAPTER SEVEN

THE ROLE OF CAREGIVERS AND FAMILY SUPPORT

RESPONSIBILITIES AND CHALLENGES OF CAREGIVING

Caregiving for someone with Alzheimer's disease involves a range of responsibilities that require both physical and emotional dedication. Primary tasks include managing daily activities such as meal preparation, personal hygiene, and medication administration.

Additionally, caregivers are responsible for ensuring the safety of the person with Alzheimer's, which might involve making modifications to the living environment, such as removing hazards and installing safety locks.

This role demands constant vigilance and adaptability, as Alzheimer's disease progresses, and the needs of the person may change rapidly.

The challenges faced by caregivers can be considerable. The emotional strain is significant, as caregivers often deal with the stress of seeing their loved one's cognitive decline. They may also experience feelings of isolation due to the demanding nature of caregiving, which can limit their social interactions and personal time. Practical challenges include managing complex healthcare needs, coordinating with various medical professionals, and dealing with financial burdens associated with long-term care. Balancing these responsibilities while maintaining one's health and well-being can be overwhelming.

TECHNIQUES FOR EFFECTIVE CAREGIVING

Effective caregiving for individuals with Alzheimer's disease requires a combination of patience, communication, and structured routines. Establishing a consistent daily routine helps reduce confusion and anxiety for the person with Alzheimer's, providing them with a sense of stability. Caregivers should focus on clear, simple instructions and use visual aids to enhance understanding. Techniques such as breaking tasks into smaller, manageable steps can make daily activities more achievable and less stressful for both the caregiver and the individual receiving care.

Employing strategies to manage challenging behaviors is also crucial. This includes understanding and anticipating triggers for agitation or aggression and employing de-escalation techniques, such as redirecting attention or using soothing language. It's beneficial for caregivers to engage in positive reinforcement and offer encouragement to reinforce desired behaviors. Creating a calm and structured environment can significantly reduce the frequency and intensity of behavioral outbursts.

IMPORTANCE OF CAREGIVER SELF-CARE

Self-care is a vital aspect of caregiving that is often overlooked. Caregivers must prioritize their health to maintain the stamina needed for their demanding role. Regular exercise, a balanced diet, and sufficient sleep are essential for physical well-being. Engaging in activities that provide relaxation and enjoyment, such as hobbies or socializing with friends, helps alleviate stress and prevent burnout. Setting aside time for oneself is crucial to sustain the ability to provide effective care.

Mental and emotional self-care is equally important. Caregivers should seek support through counseling or support groups where they can share their experiences and receive guidance. Recognizing and addressing feelings of anxiety, depression, or exhaustion is necessary for maintaining emotional health. By taking care of their own needs, caregivers can better manage the demands of their role and provide more compassionate and effective care to their loved ones.

RESOURCES AND SUPPORT NETWORKS

Utilizing available resources and support networks can significantly ease the caregiving process.

Local Alzheimer's associations and support groups offer valuable information, emotional support, and practical advice. These organizations often provide educational materials, workshops, and caregiver training to help manage various aspects of Alzheimer's care. Connecting with these resources can offer both guidance and a sense of community.

Additionally, online forums and social media groups can serve as platforms for sharing experiences and advice with other caregivers. These networks can be a source of practical tips and emotional support from individuals who understand the challenges firsthand.

Government programs and non-profit organizations may also provide financial assistance, respite care, and other services to support caregivers in their roles.

COMMUNICATING WITH HEALTHCARE PROFESSIONALS

Effective communication with healthcare professionals is critical in managing Alzheimer's disease.

Caregivers should maintain regular appointments with doctors and specialists to monitor the progression of the disease and adjust care plans as needed. Preparing detailed notes about the person's symptoms, changes in behavior, and medication responses can help facilitate more productive discussions during medical consultations.

Caregivers need to advocate for the needs of their loved ones, asking questions and expressing concerns clearly. Building a collaborative relationship with healthcare providers ensures that all aspects of care are addressed comprehensively. Understanding treatment options, medication side effects, and potential interventions can help caregivers make informed decisions and better support the well-being of the person with Alzheimer's.

CHAPTER EIGHT

LEGAL AND FINANCIAL CONSIDERATIONS

PLANNING FOR FUTURE CARE NEEDS

Planning for future care needs begins with an assessment of the individual's current and anticipated requirements. This involves evaluating their daily living activities, medical needs, and personal preferences.

Engage with healthcare professionals to develop a comprehensive care plan that outlines the type of assistance required, whether it's in-home care, adult day services, or residential facilities. This plan should be flexible to accommodate changes in the individual's condition and preferences over time.

Next, consider legal and financial preparations for future care. This includes discussing and documenting the preferences for end-of-life care and identifying potential caregivers or facilities. Establish legal documents such as advance directives or living wills to communicate medical wishes. Financially, explore long-term care insurance options and assess personal savings or assets that may be used to fund care services. Ensure that the care plan integrates seamlessly with these financial strategies to avoid unexpected expenses.

Lastly, maintain regular reviews and updates of the care plan to reflect any changes in health status or personal preferences. Regularly consulting with healthcare providers and financial advisors will help adapt the plan to meet evolving needs. Stay informed about new care options and resources that may enhance the quality of care and address any emerging needs or concerns effectively.

MANAGING FINANCES AND LEGAL DOCUMENTS

Managing finances and legal documents involves organizing and overseeing financial resources to ensure they are used effectively for care needs. Start by creating a detailed budget that includes projected costs for medical care, daily living expenses, and potential long-term care. Track all income sources, expenses, and savings to maintain a clear financial picture. Employ financial tools or software to help manage and monitor these aspects efficiently.

Legal documents must be prepared and kept up-to-date to facilitate decision-making and protect financial interests. This includes establishing a durable power of attorney for financial matters, which allows a trusted individual to manage finances on behalf of the person with Alzheimer's. Additionally, set up a will or trust to outline how assets should be distributed and appoint a guardian if necessary.

These documents help ensure that financial decisions align with the individual's wishes and legal requirements.

Regularly review and update these documents and financial plans as circumstances change. Ensure that all relevant parties, including family members and legal representatives, are aware of and understand the arrangements. This proactive management helps prevent potential conflicts and ensures that financial and legal matters are handled according to the individual's preferences and needs.

UNDERSTANDING INSURANCE AND BENEFITS

Understanding insurance and benefits requires a thorough review of available policies and how they can support care needs. Start by assessing existing health insurance policies to determine what is covered under different plans, including home care, medical treatments, and long-term care services. Contact insurance providers to clarify coverage details and ensure that the policy meets current and anticipated needs.

Explore additional benefits such as government programs, including Medicaid and Medicare, which may offer financial assistance for various care services. Understand the eligibility criteria and application processes for these programs to maximize available benefits.

Also, investigate any veterans' benefits or community-based resources that may provide additional support or financial aid.

Keep documentation of all insurance policies and benefit plans organized and readily accessible. Regularly review and adjust coverage as needed to ensure that it continues to meet the evolving care needs.

Consulting with an insurance specialist or benefits advisor can provide valuable guidance in navigating complex insurance and benefit systems.

LEGAL RIGHTS AND PROTECTIONS FOR INDIVIDUALS WITH ALZHEIMER'S

Legal rights and protections for individuals with Alzheimer's are crucial in ensuring their safety and dignity. Begin by understanding the rights afforded under laws such as the Americans with Disabilities Act (ADA), which protects against discrimination in various settings, including employment and public services.

This law ensures that individuals with Alzheimer's have access to necessary accommodations and support.

Ensure that the individual's legal rights are respected in care settings by advocating for appropriate care standards and ensuring that their preferences and decisions are honored. Familiarize yourself with guardianship or conservatorship processes if a legal representative is needed to make decisions on behalf of the person with Alzheimer's. This involves navigating court procedures and demonstrating the need for legal oversight to protect the individual's well-being.

Stay informed about advocacy organizations and support groups that focus on Alzheimer's disease. These resources can guide legal rights and offer support in addressing any concerns or disputes related to care and treatment. Engaging with these organizations can help ensure that the individual's rights are upheld and their quality of life is maintained.

RESOURCES FOR LEGAL AND FINANCIAL ADVICE

Accessing resources for legal and financial advice involves connecting with professionals who specialize in Alzheimer's care and related financial planning. Start by consulting with an elder law attorney who can guide estate planning, legal protections, and guardianship issues. They can help draft necessary legal documents and navigate complex legal scenarios specific to Alzheimer's care.

Additionally, seek advice from financial planners who have experience in managing long-term care expenses. They can assist in creating a financial strategy that addresses current needs and future costs, including investment options, budgeting, and accessing government benefits. Ensure that the planner understands the nuances of Alzheimer's care to provide tailored financial solutions.

Explore local and national resources, such as Alzheimer's Association chapters and caregiver support networks, which often offer workshops, counseling, and referral services. These resources can connect you with legal and financial advisors who have expertise in Alzheimer's care and help you stay informed about best practices and available support.

CHAPTER NINE

LIVING WITH ALZHEIMER'S DISEASE

ADAPTING TO CHANGES IN LIFESTYLE

Adjusting to a diagnosis of Alzheimer's disease requires significant lifestyle modifications. One of the first steps is to create a structured daily routine that minimizes confusion and provides a sense of stability. This can be achieved by setting up consistent meal times, regular exercise, and structured activities, which help the individual, maintain a sense of normalcy.

Simplifying tasks and breaking them into smaller, manageable steps can also alleviate frustration and confusion.

Another key aspect is modifying the living environment to accommodate changing needs. This may involve installing safety features like grab bars and non-slip mats in bathrooms and using clear, simple labels on cupboards and drawers.

Keeping the living space clutter-free can help reduce the risk of accidents and create a more navigable environment. Adapting the home in this way helps individuals with Alzheimer's maintain independence and reduce the likelihood of falls or injuries.

Additionally, incorporating adaptive technologies can assist in managing daily life. This includes using reminder systems or apps to help with appointments, medication schedules, and daily tasks. Technology can also facilitate communication with caregivers and loved ones, providing reassurance and support. By embracing these tools, individuals with Alzheimer's and their families can better manage the changes that come with the disease.

ENSURING SAFETY AND COMFORT

Ensuring safety in a home affected by Alzheimer's involves implementing several practical measures. First, it's essential to assess the home for potential hazards, such as sharp edges, electrical outlets, or stairs without handrails, and make necessary adjustments. Installing safety locks on cabinets and doors can prevent access to dangerous items while using motion-sensor lights can help prevent falls at night.

Comfort can be enhanced by creating a calm and familiar environment. Using personal items such as family photos and cherished objects can help provide a sense of continuity and security.

Comfortable furniture, appropriate bedding, and a quiet, well-lit living space contribute to a more relaxing atmosphere. Maintaining a consistent room temperature and addressing any sensory needs, such as noise or light sensitivity, further ensures a comfortable living environment.

Additionally, considering the individual's specific needs and preferences is crucial for their comfort. This includes accommodating any dietary restrictions or preferences and providing options for activities that align with their interests. Regular check-ins with healthcare providers and adjustments based on their feedback can also ensure that the person's physical and emotional well-being is continuously supported.

ENGAGING IN MEANINGFUL ACTIVITIES

Engaging individuals with Alzheimer's in meaningful activities is essential for their cognitive and emotional health. Activities should be tailored to their abilities and interests, focusing on tasks that are enjoyable and stimulating. Simple, repetitive activities such as gardening, drawing, or listening to music can provide a sense of accomplishment and joy, while also reducing anxiety and agitation.

It's beneficial to integrate familiar routines and hobbies into their daily life, as these activities can evoke positive memories and maintain cognitive function. Involving the person in household tasks, such as sorting laundry or setting the table, can also help them feel useful and engaged. Activities that promote social interaction, like joining support groups or participating in community events, can further enhance their quality of life.

Additionally, creating a daily schedule that includes a mix of physical, cognitive, and social activities helps maintain balance and prevent boredom. Regularly reviewing and adjusting the activity plan based on the individual's responses ensures that the activities remain relevant and engaging. By prioritizing their interests and abilities, caregivers can foster a more fulfilling and enjoyable daily experience.

BUILDING A SUPPORT NETWORK

Building a strong support network is crucial for both the individual with Alzheimer's and their caregivers. Start by connecting with local support groups and organizations that offer resources, education, and emotional support. These groups provide valuable opportunities for sharing experiences, learning new coping strategies, and receiving practical advice from others facing similar challenges.

Engaging family members, friends, and neighbors in the caregiving process can also help alleviate some of the emotional and physical burden.

Clear communication about the needs and preferences of the person with Alzheimer's ensures that everyone involved understands their role and responsibilities. Regular meetings with the support network can facilitate coordination and provide a forum for discussing any concerns or adjustments.

Additionally, seeking professional support from healthcare providers, social workers, or counselors can guide managing the disease and accessing community resources. These professionals can offer personalized advice, connect caregivers with additional services, and help navigate complex decisions related to care and support. Building and maintaining a robust support network strengthens the overall caregiving process and enhances the well-being of everyone involved.

PLANNING FOR END-OF-LIFE CARE

Planning for end-of-life care is a critical aspect of managing Alzheimer's disease, ensuring that the individual's wishes and needs are respected.

Begin by discussing and documenting preferences for medical treatment, including any advance directives or living wills. This allows for clear guidance on their desired level of intervention and comfort measures as the disease progresses.

It's important to explore and discuss options for palliative and hospice care with healthcare providers. These services focus on providing comfort and support rather than curative treatments, aiming to improve the quality of life in the later stages of the disease. Understanding the available options and making decisions in advance can help ensure that the individual's care aligns with their values and preferences.

Additionally, organizing practical aspects such as legal and financial matters is essential for a smooth transition. This includes updating wills, power of attorney, and any other legal documents related to health care and estate planning.

CHAPTER TEN

FAQS

WHAT ARE THE EARLY SIGNS OF ALZHEIMER'S DISEASE?

Early signs of Alzheimer's disease often include subtle memory loss, particularly difficulty remembering recent events or conversations. Individuals may frequently ask the same questions or become confused about the time or place.

Changes in judgment and decision-making are also common; for example, a person may struggle with managing finances or planning meals. These early symptoms can be so mild that they might be dismissed as normal aging.

Additionally, Alzheimer's may cause difficulties with familiar tasks and routines. An individual might forget how to perform tasks they previously did easily, such as operating household appliances or following a recipe.

Spatial disorientation can also occur, leading to getting lost in familiar places or having trouble understanding spatial relationships.

Language problems are another early sign. This might include difficulty finding the right words, repeating themselves, or having trouble following or joining conversations. These signs often gradually become more pronounced and can interfere with daily functioning and interactions with others.

ARE THERE ANY LIFESTYLE CHANGES THAT CAN REDUCE THE RISK OF DEVELOPING ALZHEIMER'S?

Lifestyle changes that may reduce the risk of developing Alzheimer's include adopting a heart-healthy diet, such as the Mediterranean diet, which emphasizes fruits, vegetables, whole grains, and healthy fats. Regular physical activity is also crucial; activities like walking, swimming, or cycling can improve cardiovascular health and support brain function.

Engaging in mental stimulation through activities like reading, puzzles, and learning new skills can keep the brain active and potentially delay the onset of symptoms. Social interaction is equally important; maintaining strong social connections and participating in group activities can enhance cognitive reserve and reduce the risk of cognitive decline.

Additionally, managing chronic conditions such as diabetes, hypertension, and high cholesterol can lower the risk of Alzheimer's. Ensuring adequate sleep, reducing stress, and avoiding smoking and excessive alcohol consumption are also beneficial for overall brain health.

HOW IS ALZHEIMER'S DISEASE DIAGNOSED?

Diagnosing Alzheimer's disease involves a comprehensive assessment, starting with a detailed medical history and a physical examination. Physicians often conduct cognitive tests to evaluate memory, problem-solving skills, and other cognitive functions.

Standard tests include the Mini-Mental State Examination (MMSE) or the Montreal Cognitive Assessment (MoCA).

Imaging studies such as MRI or CT scans are used to rule out other conditions and identify changes in brain structure that may indicate Alzheimer's. Additionally, positron emission tomography (PET) scans can be utilized to detect amyloid plaques and tau tangles, which are characteristic of Alzheimer's Disease.

A definitive diagnosis may involve a lumbar puncture (spinal tap) to analyze cerebrospinal fluid for biomarkers associated with Alzheimer's. In some cases, genetic testing may be used if there is a family history of the disease, although this is not always necessary or conclusive.

WHAT TYPES OF MEDICATIONS ARE USED TO TREAT ALZHEIMER'S, AND HOW DO THEY WORK?

Medications used to treat Alzheimer's primarily focus on managing symptoms and slowing disease progression. Cholinesterase inhibitors, such as donepezil, rivastigmine, and galantamine, work by increasing levels of acetylcholine, a neurotransmitter important for memory and learning. These drugs can help improve cognitive symptoms and daily functioning.

Another class of drugs, NMDA receptor antagonists like memantine, helps regulate the activity of glutamate, a neurotransmitter involved in learning and memory. Memantine is often prescribed in conjunction with cholinesterase inhibitors for moderate to severe Alzheimer's.

In addition to these, there are medications aimed at managing behavioral symptoms, such as depression, anxiety, or aggression that may arise in Alzheimer's patients.

Antidepressants, antipsychotics, and mood stabilizers are used selectively based on the individual's specific needs and symptoms.

HOW CAN CAREGIVERS COPE WITH THE CHALLENGES OF CARING FOR SOMEONE WITH ALZHEIMER'S?

Caregivers can manage the challenges of Alzheimer's care by establishing a structured routine to provide stability and reduce confusion for the person with the disease. Creating a predictable daily schedule, including regular meal times, activities, and rest periods, can help minimize agitation and improve the individual's sense of security.

Support systems are essential for caregivers. Seeking help from family members, friends, or support groups can provide emotional support and practical advice. Respite care services, which offer temporary relief from caregiving duties, can also help caregivers maintain their well-being and avoid burnout.

Educating oneself about Alzheimer's and its progression helps caregivers understand what to expect and how to address various symptoms effectively.

Utilizing resources such as caregiver training programs and professional guidance can equip caregivers with strategies to handle challenging behaviors and ensure a better quality of life for both the caregiver and the person with Alzheimer's.

www.ingramcontent.com/pod-product-compliance
Lightning Source LLC
Chambersburg PA
CBHW070205230526
45471CB00002B/829